How to Treat Stress and Anxiety

Naturally and Effectively

Ryder Management Inc.

Epigraph

"Study nature; Love nature; Stay close to nature; it will never fail you.
Frank Lloyd Wright

"Your body's ability to heal is greater than anyone has permitted you to believe."
Unknown

.

Table of Contents

Introduction 1

Stress vs Anxiety 1

    Nervines 3

    Adaptogens 3

Ashwagandha (Withania somnifera).........................5

Astragalus (Astragalus Membranaceus) 7

Blue Vervain (Verbena hastate) 8

Catnip (Nepeta cataria)..9

Chamomile (Matricaria chamomilla) 11

Dream Herb (Calea zacatechichi)...........................12

Eleuthero Root (Eleutherococcus senticosis)........13

Golden Root (Rhodiola Rosea) 14

Hibiscus 15

Holy Basil (Ocimum sanctum) 17

Hops (Humulus lupulus)..18

Honeybush (Cyclopia spp)......................................20

Lapacho (Tabebuia impetiginosa) 21

Lavender (Lavendula)..22

Lemon Balm (Melissa officinalis) 23

Motherwort (Leonurus cardiac)..............................25

Mulungu (Erythrina mulungu) 26

Passionflower (Passiflora incarnata)......................27

Rooibos (Aspalathus linearis)..................................29

Schisandra Berries (Schisandra chinensis) 31

Skullcap (Scutellaria lateriflora) 32

St John's Wort (Hypericum perforatum)..................33

Valerian (Valeriana officinalis) 34

Wormwood (Artemisia absinthium) 36

Closing Remarks...38

About the Author...39

References and Sources.......................................40

Introduction

When we were young, our bodies enjoyed the inherent vitality that comes with youth. As we age however, it is important to be aware of the way our mind and body reacts to everyday challenges and demands. Learning how to manage stress is a very important function of staying healthy and looking and feeling vibrant.

Did you know that there exists a unique class of healing plants, called adaptogens that are able to protect and restore our body back to a harmonious state?

Herbal medicine dates back to the beginning of time and is a common element in all traditional methods of healing including Native American, homeopathic and naturopathic, in the West along with Tibetan, Ayurvedic and Traditional Chinese Medicine (TCM), in the East.

This book includes a number of natural herbal remedies that can provide an overall calming effect on our mind and body. This calming effect is made possible from the natural compound in some herbs known as nervines. In addition, this book includes a number of herbal adaptogens that are able to restore our overall well-being and prevent, control and alleviate stress and anxiety.

It is important to deal with stress at or close to its inception in order to prevent stress from building up to anxiety. Combating and/or nipping stress in the bud will also prevent the development of more serious diseases such as cancer. The benefits of using natural herbal products provide a number of additional (and beneficial) side benefits too including vitamins, nutrients , boosting immunity and giving a general overall sense of well-being , depending on the herb of choice.

The most common method of consuming any of the herbs discussed in this book is by brewing and enjoying them in a cup of tea. Other methods include adding the powdered equivalent to your favorite juice or smoothie. To make a tea, add one teaspoon of dried herb or one tablespoon of fresh herb to a cup of boiling water and let steep for up to 15 minutes before consuming.

The purpose of this book is to provide you with information on alternative sources of remedies that can effectively help you combat and deal with stress and anxiety naturally and effectively.

Stress vs Anxiety

What is the difference between stress and anxiety?

The definition of stress according to Merriam-Webster is *"a state of mental tension and worry caused by problems in your life, work, etc.; something that causes strong feelings of worry; physical force or pressure"*. A *stressor* is anything that causes stress and can include people, places, events and objects.

Merriam-Webster defines anxiety as *"fear or nervousness about what might happen; a feeling of wanting to do something very much"*.

From the above definitions, we can infer that stress comes from the pressures we feel in life, as we are pushed by work or other tasks that seems to put undue pressure on our minds and body. Anxiety is one of the negative effects of stress. Whereas stress is caused by existing stressors, anxiety is stress that continues after the stressor is gone. Anxiety is almost always associated with a feeling of impending doom.

The stress hormone, cortisol, belongs to a class of hormones called glucocorticoids, which affect almost every organ and tissue in our body. The most important function of cortisol is to assist our body respond to stress. The amount of cortisol produced by the adrenal glands is precisely balanced. Elevated levels of cortisol can make us anxious and irritable, lead to weight gain and bone loss and deplete our energy and contribute to the risk of diabetes and heart disease. When cortisol gets too high, it elevates the "flight or fight" response, which affects our nervous system and adrenal glands. When our body is in a state of constant stress, we can age more rapidly than we otherwise should.

The plant based remedies that follow are specific classes of herbs called nervines and adaptogens and both classes have been found to be effective in reducing stress and anxiety

Nervines

Nervines are plant based remedies that specifically support and have a beneficial effect on the nervous system. These herbs are very effective in reducing stress and tension. Nervines are complimentary herbs for adaptogens and have a calming effect on the nervous system. Most can be consumed throughout the day to help maintain a calm composure.

Adaptogens

Adaptogens are a unique and rare group of plant compounds that have a beneficial and healthy effect on our adrenal system, the system responsible for managing our body's response to stress. They are called adaptogens because of their unique ability of "adapting" their function according to our body's specific need at any given time.

The first scientific paper on adaptogens was published in 1960 and was written by Dr. Israel Brekhman, a renowned Russian scientist. This first publication on adaptogens was the culmination of 15 years of scientific research on adaptogens. Dr. Brekhman coined the phrase "adaptogen" to classify naturally occurring substances found in a rare group of plants and herbs. To be considered an adaptogen, the plant must possess all of the following three characteristics:

The plant increases the body's nonspecific resistance to internal and external stimuli,

The plant is able to bring any deficiency in the body back to a state of balance; AND

The plant is absolutely safe and non-toxic.

Surprisingly, adaptogens have been used in Traditional Chinese Medicine and Indian Ayurvedic medicine for centuries as a remedy for boosting energy and resilience in the face of stress.

Following is an alphabetical listing of nervines and/or adaptogens, special plants that are able to help our bodies deal with stress and anxiety effectively, without any side effects.

Ashwagandha (Withania somnifera)

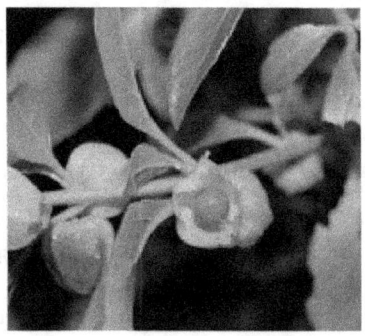

Withania somnifera, also known as Ashwagandha, Indian ginseng, or winter cherry, has long been an important herb in the Ayurvedic and indigenous medical systems. It is grown in Africa the Mediterranean and India. As an adaptogen, it helps the body fight stress by reducing the production of stress hormones that result in the fight or flight response. It also contains a chemical compound called ashwagandholine alkaloid, which has a mild relaxing and somewhat tranquilizing effect on the central nervous system.

Ashwagandha is an herb used in Ayurvedic medicine for a number of health conditions. Known by the botanical name *Withania somnifera*, it is a popular medicinal plant in South East Asia and Southern Europe. Many people use this herb for general vitality, although the effects are not similar to ginseng. Rather than providing restless energy like ginseng, ashwagandha often causes relaxation.

Withania somnifera is widely considered the Indian ginseng. In Ayurveda, it is classified as a rasayana (rejuvenation) and expected to promote physical and mental health, rejuvenate the body in debilitated conditions and increase longevity.

Ashwagandha is used to treat a number of disorders that affect human health including central nervous system (CNS) disorders, particularly epilepsy; stress and neurodegenerative diseases such as Parkinson's and Alzheimer's disorders; tardive dyskinesia (involuntary facial movements) , cerebral ischemia (brain disorders), and even the management of drug addiction withdrawal. However, the most revered use of this King of Herbs is its ability to reduce stress and perhaps aid in sleep.

Decoction: Make a mild decoction of 1 teaspoon of dried root to each cup of water. Drink a small portion 3 times daily over a 2 to 3 week period to start feeling the effects. Powdered root can also be infused with hot milk and honey or added to smoothies, beginning with 1/4 teaspoon and increasing to 1-2 teaspoons per day slowly.

Astragalus (Astragalus Membranaceus)

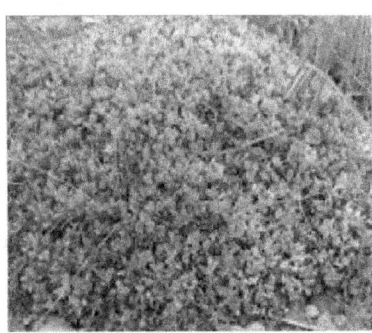

Astragalus (Astragalus membranaceus) is a perennial plant that is able to grow up to three feet in height. It is native to the northern and eastern regions of China as well as Mongolia and Korea and belongs to the legume family, *Fabaceae.* The root is the medicinal part of the plant and is usually harvested from plants that are at least four years old.

Astragalus has been used in Traditional Chinese Medicine for centuries. It is considered an adaptogen and is often combined with various other adaptogens to enhance the ability to heal a particular disease. For example, when Astragalus is combined with Schisandra berries, the concoction is very effective in reversing cirrhosis of the liver.

Astragalus has antibacterial and anti-inflammatory properties as well as antioxidants. Astragalus has been used to treat mental, emotional and physical stress and anxiety; colds and flus; diabetes; fatigue; heart disease; hepatitis; kidney and liver disease.

The recommended dose is to make a decoction of strong boiled tea by adding 1-2 teaspoons of dried root powder to 12 oz. of boiling water and let sit for 15-20 minutes to allow the herb to extract in the hot water.

Blue Vervain (Verbena hastate)

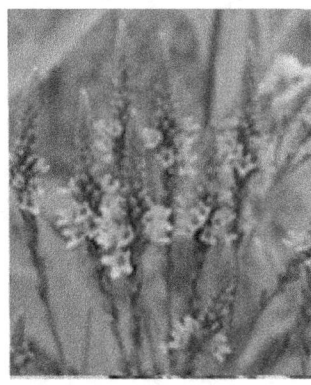

Blue Vervain (also referred to as verbena) is a creeping perennial of the mint family, Lamiaceae. However, "phylogenetic studies" in the 1990's have debated the taxonomic classification of numerous species and as a result, moved V. hastate (the scientific name of Blue Vervain) to the Verbenaceae family. It is classified as a wildflower that can grow from two to five feet tall. It spreads through rhizomes, similar to mint. (This means that its roots spread underground).

Blue Vervain is a hardy herb that is native to all areas of North America with the exception of the Canadian province of Alberta, (according to the US Database on plants).

The "ethnobotany" of this herb in the west is its ability to treat depression. However, it is also effective with treating fevers, stomach cramps, coughs and headaches. Externally, it can be used to treat acne and cuts. The Dakota tribe (First People in North America)

One of the most prominent uses for Vervain is in a tea due to its natural ability in reducing feelings of anxiety and boosting overall mood. Blue Vervain has a bitter taste and consequently, most animals, with the exception of the cottontail rabbit, avoid it.

Due to its bitter taste, it is necessary to sweeten a tea made with this herb with honey.

Catnip (Nepeta cataria)

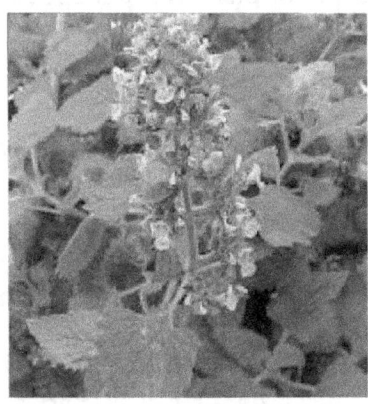

All cats, by nature, love catnip. Did you know that there are a number of medicinal properties in this plant for cat owners too? In other words, cats and cat owners can both benefit from this nervine herb.

Nepeta cataria (catnip, catnep, catswort, or catmint) is a species of the genus Nepeta in the large Lamiaceae family (also known as the Mint family). It is native to much of Asia and Europe, and now widely naturalized elsewhere. The common names may also refer to the genus as a whole. It is a 50–100 cm tall herbaceous perennial that resembles mint in appearance. It can appear to have greyish-green leaves; the flowers are white with a purple hue.

Nepeta cataria is thought to have originated in Europe and Asia. The herb was transported to various parts of the globe and can now be found growing wild in parts of Africa and North America, as well as Europe and Asia. In

The plant can grow to a height of about 3 feet and looks similar to the mint plant. The leaves are green and may show a gray colored tinge, the tightly clustered flowers are purple and may have small white or pale lavender spots.

Catnip has a history of being used as a food, garden plant, and for other purposes. The essential oil can be used as a natural insecticide. The leaves can be used to add flavor to sauces, soups and stews, they can also be chewed to reduce toothache.

The dried leaves, seeds or powdered roots can be made into herbal tea. Catnip tea has been has been found to have an anticholinergic effect.

The main chemical that causes psychoactive effects when a person uses Nepeta cataria is nepetalactone. It has antibacterial properties and is a mild sedative that can reduce fever, nervous and muscular spasms, or convulsions.

Usage: Boil 2 tablespoons of dried Catnip in 3-4 cups (800-1000 ml) of filtered water. Let it rest for 15 minutes. Add honey as an optional flavoring to sweeten.

Chamomile (Matricaria chamomilla)

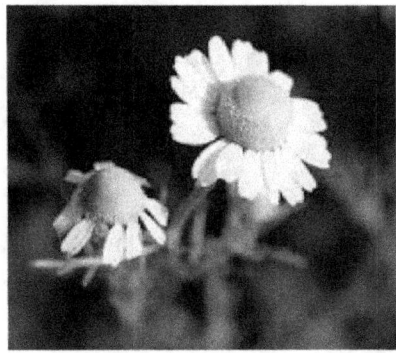

Chamomile (Matricaria chamomilla) has a long history of medicinal use. It is a flowering plant that is scientifically classified as belonging to the daisy family, Asteraceae. It is a nervine herb that is very effective and useful for relieving headaches, general pain and mental stress. It has a long history of use in calming the nervous system and as a support for digestion.

Chamomile helps to relax and organize a group of nerves that affect the upper gastrointestinal function. It relaxes the stomach and contains anti-inflammatory, anti-spasmodic and anti-bacterial properties which all help the body combat stress. It is a relaxing tea for relief from anxiety, upset stomach, irritability, nervous headaches, insomnia and irritable bowel syndrome.

Organic Chamomile tea is widely available in tea bags.

Dream Herb (Calea zacatechichi)

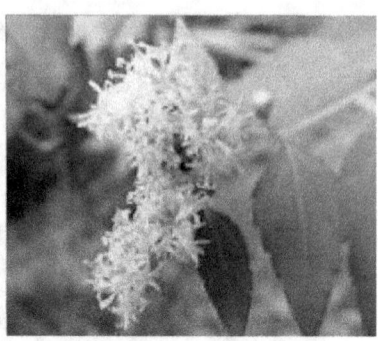

Calea zacatechichi, also known as Dream Herb, Leaf of God, and Bitter Grass, is a plant used by the indigenous Chontal of the Mexican state of Oaxaca for one iromancy (a form of divination based on dreams.) The plant naturally occurs from southern Mexico to northern Costa Rica. There are currently two reported varieties, one being extremely bitter and the other non-bitter.

Calea zacatechichi (Dream Herb/Leaf of God) is a plant used by the Chontal Indians of Mexico to obtain divinatory messages through dreaming. Clinical studies show that ingestion of the plant produces a light hypnotic state with a decrease of both deep slow-wave sleep and REM periods. Traditionally the plant was drank as a tea while a cigarette made from the Calea was smoked before bed, bringing relaxation and fluidity to mind and body, ushering in an easy and deep sleep during which the dreamer will find the gates to the dreamscape gently opened.

Calea tea: Add 3 grams of dried herb to a cup of hot water. Let it soak for 15 minutes. After filtering increase the flavor with honey.

Eleuthero Root (Eleutherococcus senticosis)

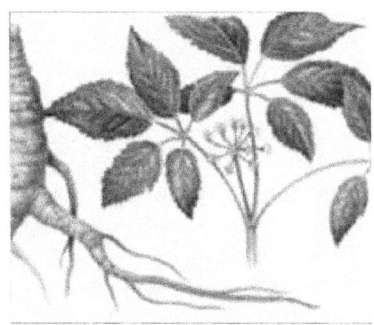

Eleuthero Root (Eleutherococcus senticosis) is a woody shrub from the Araliaceae family. It is native to China, Korea, japan and Russia and was formerly called Siberian Ginseng, a name banned in the United States by the Ginseng Labeling Act of 2002.

Eleuthero is a top rated adaptogenic herb which can enhance the body's natural ability to adapt to stress, while supporting mental endurance and metabolic efficiency.

Despite its former name – Siberian Ginseng, it is completely different from Asian ginseng (Panax ginseng) and American ginseng (Panax quinquefolius). Eleuthero is widely used in Russia as an adaptogen.

The benefits of Eleuthero include anti-anxiety and extra energy; increased circulation which helps in restoring memory, concentration and mental clarity; anti-fatigue; and an effective immune booster. This herb is also beneficial to the liver and it contains antiviral properties.

Golden Root (Rhodiola Rosea)

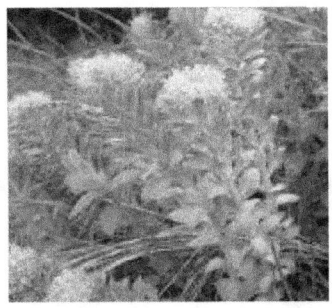

Rhodiola rosea, also called Golden Root, is an adaptogen that grows in the Arctic regions of eastern Siberia. It is a powerful antidepressant that restores inner reserves. This herb is a popular plant in traditional medical systems in Eastern Europe and Asia. Russians have drunk Rhodiola tea for centuries as an energy booster. Russian and Chinese scientists have researched the benefits of the root for several decades.

Dozens of species of Rhodiola plants grow wild in nature. The root has a reputation for stimulating the nervous system, fighting depression, enhancing work performance, decreasing fatigue, and reducing high altitude sickness. This herb has been categorized as an adaptogen by Russian researchers due to its observed ability to increase resistance to a variety of chemical, biological, and physical stressors.

Rhodiola rosea contains a phyto chemical called salisdroside that helps combat anxiety and aging. It suppresses the production of cortisol and increases levels of stress-resistant proteins. Studies show that it also restores normal eating and sleep patterns, combats mental and physical fatigue and protects against oxidative stress, radiation and exposure to toxic chemicals.

Rhodiola also protects the heart and liver, increases the use of oxygen, improves memory and focus and may even extend longevity.

For a tea, soak 5 grams of Rhodiola Rosea in one cup of hot water for 4 hours. It can be consumed after filtering and adding optional flavorings such as cinnamon, nutmeg, and honey.

Hibiscus

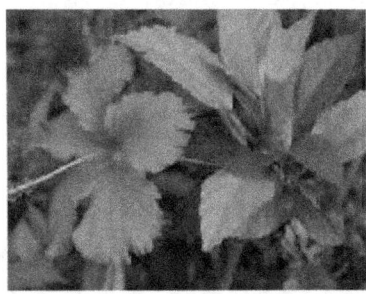

Hibiscus is a genus of flowering plants in the mallow family, Malvaceae. It is a large family containing several hundred species that are native to warm-temperate, subtropical and tropical regions throughout the world. Member species are often noted for their showy flowers and are commonly known simply as hibiscus, or less widely known as rose mallow

Hibiscus tea is made from the Hibiscus; it is the sepals of the flower that are used to make the herbal tea. In this tea there is no caffeine so has no side effects.

It acts as a natural antioxidant. Antioxidants fight with the free radicals in the body. These also boost cell growth, immune system and decrease the risk of cancer and cataracts. It reduces premature aging. Hibiscus tea also controls the blood pressure, liver disorders and high cholesterol. Hibiscus tea thus reduces the chances of heart diseases. It lowers the blood pressure so people having low blood pressure should not consume it. Hibiscus tea is also act as antispasmodic. Thus it reduces the muscle cramps, stomach cramps and even the menstrual cramps. It is also very effective in losing weight. The enzyme called amylase breaks down the starch and sugar in the body, thus helping you to reduce weight. Therefore you can take a sip of hibiscus tea after meal as this will lower the absorption of carbohydrates. This further will help you in reducing weight. Hibiscus tea strengthens the immune system as it contains great amount of vitamin C. Vitamin C is beneficial for immune system. So your body will fight against fever and flu more strongly with firm immune system.

To make hibiscus tea:

Boil 2-3 cups of water in a saucepan and turn off the heat. Add two tablespoon of dried petals in boiled water. For a more exotic taste put 1 or 2 cinnamon sticks into water. Cover it and keep it for 15 to 20 minutes. Do not keep it beyond 20 minutes as this will lead to bitterness. In case you want strong tea then add more flower to the water. Strain the tea. Add lemon and honey for flavor if desired but without flavoring hibiscus tea has a strong and fresh sour taste.

Warning:

Hibiscus tea affects estrogen level. Also person who has gone for the hormone replacement therapy and using birth control pills should avoid it. Pregnant and breast-feeding mothers should not take it. People taking anti-cancer drugs should not take it.

Holy Basil (Ocimum sanctum)

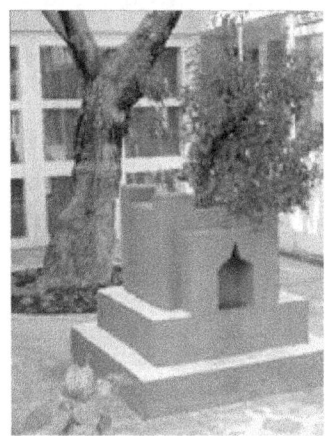

Holy Basil (also called Tulsi and Tulsi Holy Basil) is known in India as the Queen of Herbs or the "elixir of anti-aging" in Ayurveda medicine. Its botanical name is Ocimum sanctum and is from the Lamiaceae or mint family.

Tulsi functions as an adaptogen, enhancing the body's natural response to physical and emotional stress by helping it function optimally during stressful times.

Holy Basil (Ocimum sanctum) is not the same as sweet basil used in cooking spaghetti sauce.

Tulsi Holy Basil has a number of adaptogenic properties that help combat stress. In fact, modern research has shown that Tulsi prevents elevated levels of cortisol. Tulsi also has anti-bacterial properties and helps prevent cancer, heart disease and diabetes. The leaves are considered a nerve tonic and also sharpen the memory.

The daily use of Tulsi leaf and flowers is believed to balance the chakras or energetic centers of the body, and to bring joy and virtue.

Holy Basil is available in tea form from a number of health food and homeopath stores. My most favorite blend of Holy Basil tea is available at TrulyOrganicFoods.com.

Hops (Humulus lupulus)

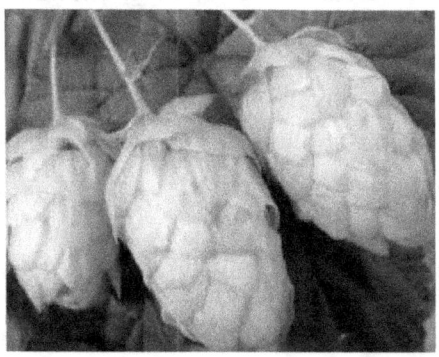

Although hops are the main ingredient in beer, hops also possess medicinal properties, whose health benefits were widely used in traditional and herbal healing where it is known as an entheogen. Hops are also considered a nervine.

Hops are a vigorous, herbaceous climbing perennial that is native to Europe and Asia. Hops belong to the same family as Cannabis sativa, which is Cannabaceae.

Hops have traditionally been used for a variety of health benefits which has recently been confirmed through scientific research. Among the plethora of health benefits, the most prominent include sleep inducer and relaxation, anti-inflammatory, antioxidant and anti-anxiety. Hops have also been found to contain estrogen like chemicals, making it beneficial for medical conditions associated with hormonal changes.

Hops have also been found to contain anti-cancer fighting benefits. The Phytotherapy Research, November, 2008 edition reported that xanthohumol, a compound in hops, showed inhibitory effects on human hepatocellular carcinoma cell lines (liver cancer). In addition, the Journal of Experimental and Molecular Pathology (April 2012) reported a study that the bitter acids from hops exhibit anti-fibrogenic effects on hepatic stellate cells in vitro. This means that hops contain healing properties that benefit chronic liver diseases such as cirrhosis.

Hops tea has many health advantages that come from the secondary plant metabolites including flavonoids. These health benefits include a variety of natural ways to help heal and rejuvenate the body.

As natural and herbal forms of treatment begin finding their way back into the hands of the general public, herbal teas and remedies such as hops tea have been securing a place on the shelves of more homes than ever before.

Hops tea has a number of external benefits and uses as well as internal. For cuts, burns, bruises, bug bites and small scrapes, to speed healing and to relieve pain and discomfort, use a small cloth, dipped in cooled hops tea and apply to the wound. Rinsing hair with cooled hops tea also relieves dry itchy scalps.

Honeybush (Cyclopia spp)

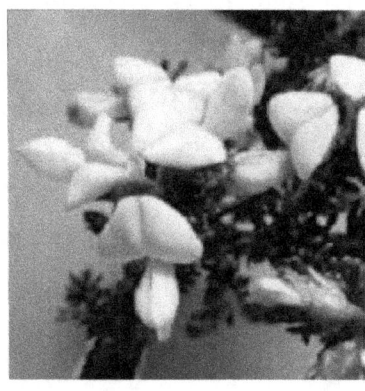

Honeybush tea is brewed from the honey-scented flowers, leaves and stems of various species of the South African Honeybush shrub, it is known scientifically as Cyclopia. Honeybush is from the legume family Fabaceae and shares many similarities with rooibos.

South African herbalists have long valued this herb for its medicinal properties. Today, many of these properties have been confirmed by modern medical research.

Honeybush is a healthy, caffeine-free red tea that contains Vitamin C, potassium, calcium and magnesium. With a mildly sweet taste, exquisite honey aroma, and unique wellness benefits, it makes a delicious hot or cold beverage. Honeybush tea is a natural source of many antioxidants, including major phenolic compounds. Phenolic compounds play a significant role in protecting the immune system from oxidative stress, which could damage cells. The phenolic compounds in Honeybush tea are able to reduce inflammation and prevent the development of chronic inflammatory diseases. Honeybush tea is also effective in relieving menopausal symptoms in women. According to the newest studies Honeybush tea prevents the body from storing more fat and may even help breakdown existing fat.

Usage: Brewing the tea increases the antioxidant value, flavor, and color of the tea and Honeybush tea never gets bitter. Honeybush can also be made in a teapot and then poured through a strainer, or by using a tea ball or tea filter. Use 1 teaspoon of tea leaves or one tea bag per cup.

Lapacho (Tabebuia impetiginosa)

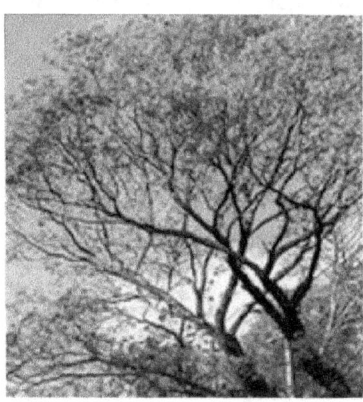

Lapacho is an evergreen tree that is native to South America. The inner bark and wood of the tree has been used medicinally for centuries for a variety of health purposes.

As an herbal tea, it does not contain caffeine, and it is rich in essential vitamins and minerals that help maintain health and vitality. Lapacho tea, for example, contains iron, calcium, magnesium, manganese, iodine, boron and barium. The active constituents of Lapacho are thought to be the two compounds lapachol and beta-lapachone, as well as their derivatives. Lapachol and beta-lapachone, demonstrate anti-inflammatory, antimalarial and immune-modulating activity. Lapacho has antimicrobial properties and may therefore help to kill bacteria, fungi, viruses and parasites. Lapacho tea also demonstrates antioxidant activity and may help to prevent free radical-induced damage to your cells and DNA. Lapacho is also used to help reduce pain and treat inflammatory disorders In addition, the tea is purported to promote the healing of boils, ulcers and other wounds. Lapacho has blood-thinning effects and slows clotting. Excessive amounts of Lapacho tea, exceeding 1.5 g of bark and wood per day, may cause bleeding and vomiting. Pregnant women thus should not take Lapacho, and to be on the safe side, breastfeeding women should not take it either.

Uses: Take 2 teaspoons of Lapacho tree bark, add 1 liter of boiling water and boil on a very low fire for 5-10 minutes. Then, remove the tea from heat and leave for 10-20 minutes to infuse. You can prepare Lapacho tea in advance and store in in your fridge: it will not lose its nutritional value for a couple of days.

Lavender (Lavendula)

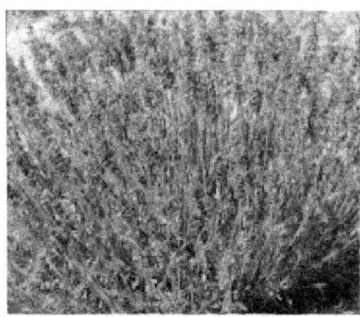

Lavender is a flowering plant belonging to the mint family, Lamiaceae. It is said to be native to the "Old World" (Africa, Europe and Asia) but is grown extensively the world over.

There are approximately 39 species of lavender and the genus includes both annual and perennial plants, shrub-like plants, subshrubs and small shrubs.

A calming nervine herb that is used extensively in aromatherapy.

Although not commonly used as tea in the west, lavender tea is prepared by adding two teaspoons of flowers in a mixture of boiled water and steeped for approximately five minutes.

The benefits of drinking lavender tea provide a number of health benefits including anti-anxiety, anti-depressant, mood stabilizing and pain relief. It also is beneficial as a sedative for those suffering from insomnia.

The health benefits of consuming lavender tea is far reaching and even extends to our gastrointestinal system. Lavender tea has been found to be effective with issues such as colic, bowel infections and flatulence.

Unsweetened lavender tea has also been used as an effective hair rinse for problems associated with hair loss. It also helps to alleviate dry scalp and dandruff too.

Lemon Balm (Melissa officinalis)

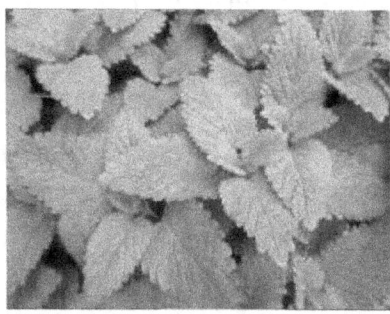

Lemon balm is a perennial herb belonging to the mint family, Lamiaceae. This nervine herb was dedicated to the goddess Diana, and was used medicinally be the Greeks for thousands of years.

Lemon balm has many health benefits, the most widely of which is a remedy for sleep disorders, stress and nervous agitation. It was traditionally used for bronchial inflammation, earaches, fever, headaches, high blood pressure, influenza, palpitations and vomiting. A tea made from the leaves of Lemon balm is known to relieve menstrual cramps and PMS as well.

During the Middle Ages, lemon balm was used to soothe nervous tension, to dress wounds, as a cure for toothaches, skin eruptions, mad dog bites, crooked necks and morning sickness associated with pregnancy. It was even used as a remedy to cure baldness.

The European Scientific Cooperative on Phytotherapy (ESCOP) lists the internal use of lemon balm for restlessness, irritability and symptomatic treatment of digestive disorders. It is also said to be a treatment for herpes labialis (ESCOP, 1997).

Recent studies on lemon balm show that it is effective in treating auto-immune disorders such as Grave's Disease. The most prominent terpene native and named from this family is limonene. Limonene is a secondary plant metabolite that increases vitality and the ability to thrive.

To prove this herbs effectiveness in treating anxiety and insomnia, a current study showed that it produced an unexpected result showing that it greatly increases the ability to concentrate and perform word and picture tasks. A subsequent study from North Umbria University in England showed that students taking lemon balm were notably calmer and less stressed during exams.

This herb is very easy to grow but spreads like mint, if not contained. A tea made with fresh leaves is absolutely heavenly.

Motherwort (Leonurus cardiac)

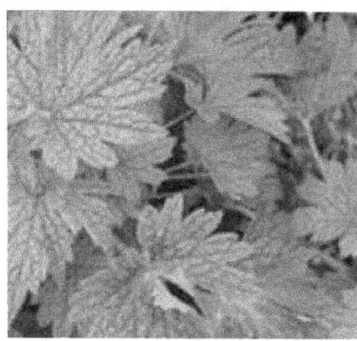

Motherwort (Leonurus cardiac) is an herbaceous perennial from the mint family, Lamiaceae. Motherwort is said to be native to Europe and Asia and was introduced to North America by colonists. It can grow up to four feet in height and produces light reddish white flowers.

Motherwort has a long history of use as a cardio tonic as well as a nervine. The effect of this plant on the nervous system is quite profound. While relaxing the nervous system it also elevates mood.

Motherwort is also found to be effective in treating anxiety, asthma, flatulence, high blood pressure, hyperthyroidism, insomnia, irregular heartbeat and menopausal symptoms.

Motherwort is very effective, when combined with blue Vervain for anxiety. Homeopaths recommend two parts motherwort to one part blue Vervain in a tea.

Mulungu (Erythrina mulungu)

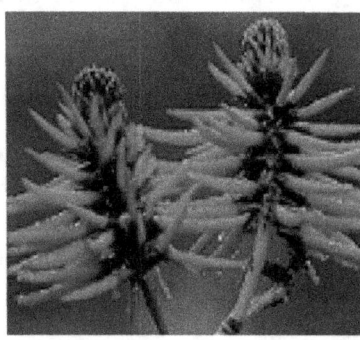

Erythrina mulungu (Mulungu) is a Brazilian ornamental tree and medicinal plant native to the cerrado and caatinga ecoregions in Brazil, South America. In Brazil mulungu has a long history of use as a natural sedative. The herb is said to be able to stabilize the central nervous system. During times of stress, this herb is able to balance and calm the nerves. The herb is also used as an antioxidant; to tone, balance and strengthen the liver.

The bark of this graceful Amazonian coral tree is a useful hypnotic sedative traditionally used for anxiety and to calm nervous tension. It is also known as an effective treatment for insomnia, rheumatism, asthma, and to strengthen the liver.

Use of Mulungu for anxiety and stress has been validated by recent studies that reveal it is able to produce an anti-anxiety effect similar to the pharmaceutical drug diazepam. Studies also show that this herb contains antibacterial, anti-inflammatory, and liver protective actions. Modern herbal medicine utilizes Mulungu to support the liver, to promote healthy sleep patterns, to strengthen the heart, and to help with drug withdrawal.

The bark of this plant contains secondary metabolites including alkaloids, flavonoids, and triterpenes.

To make Mulungu tea: add 3-5 grams of Mulungu bark to two cups of boiling water and immediately remove from heat and steep for 15-20 minutes. If the desired effect does not occur after an hour, increase the quantity of herb to 5-10 grams for your next batch.

Passionflower (Passiflora incarnata)

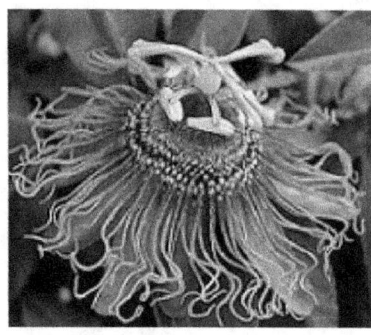

Passion Flower is a non-drowsy natural sedative that relieves nervousness, anxiety and panic attacks. This natural remedy will leave you feeling emotionally balanced by controlling emotional highs and lows.

Passionflower contains the flavone chrysin, responsible for the anti-anxiety benefits that have been shown to work similarly to the pharmaceutical Xanax (Alprazolam).

Passiflora species are native to tropical and subtropical areas of the Americas according to literature. Known for its fragrance and unique colorful flowers, passionflower was traditionally used as a calming herb. The ancient Aztecs reportedly used passionflower as a sedative and pain reliever. Today herbalists also recommend it as a sedative and antispasmodic agent.

Passionflower has been used for anxiety, insomnia, restlessness, epilepsy, and other conditions of hyperactivity, as well as high blood pressure. Low doses of passion flower tea reduce anxiety, while higher doses produce a sedative effect. T

The properties in passionflower make it useful as a soothing sleep-aid and in supporting relaxation in times of stress. Passion flower may offer benefits for management of menopause in women who either cannot or choose not to use hormone replacement therapy.

Since passionflower is a nervine, meaning that it has an effect on the nervous system, it can intensify the effects of prescription sedatives. Do not take passionflower if you are already taking prescription medication for anxiety or depression, as excessive sleepiness has been reported.

To make tea: Steep about 1 tablespoon of dried herb in 1 cup of boiling water and let steep for 10 minutes; strain and cool. For anxiety, drink 3 - 4 cups per day.

If you are experiencing sleep disorders, such as insomnia, drink one cup an hour before bed time.

The Latin name Passiflora incarnata translates as "passion made real".

Rooibos (Aspalathus linearis)

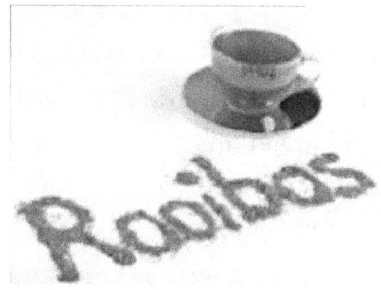

Rooibos pronounced "Roy-boss" is considered a red tea and is native to the Cape Town region of South Africa. The herbal tea made from rooibos has been a popular drink in Southern Africa for generations. Rooibos tea is a tea brewed from the plant Aspalathus linearis, and it is becoming a more popular beverage to drink in part due to its semi-sweet taste (less bitter than green and black tea) and having no caffeine content. It is also known as African red bush tea.

The vibrant amber hue comes from the natural colorants that develop during the post-harvest fermentation or oxidation process and is brought about by natural enzymes in the plant. In other words, upon harvest the leaves are green but then transcend into a gorgeous rustic shade of red when oxidized.

One of the key health benefits of rooibos tea is that it contains several minerals that are vital to health. Rooibos tea contains a wide array of antioxidants, which help to protect the body. It can improve circulation by preventing the activity of the enzyme that triggers cardiovascular disease. Drinking rooibos tea also has been known to lower blood pressure and cholesterol. It has the ability to relieve numerous abdominal ailments such as cramps, diarrhea and indigestion. Rooibos tea contains phenyl pyretic acid, which can help to improve acne, psoriasis and eczema. It also relieves nervous tension.

Current western research is showing that rooibos tea is extraordinarily rich in a wide array of antioxidants including two polyphenols called aspalathin and nothofagin which are both unique to this plant. These amazing compounds protect our bodies from the cell damaging effects of free radicals, thereby further protecting us from a host of degenerative diseases including Parkinson's disease, Alzheimer's and various forms of cancer. In fact, the Cancer Association of South Africa, after eight years of research, has now officially recognized Rooibos as a leading source of natural anti-cancer chemicals.

Similar to many other herbal teas, such as ginger tea, rooibos tea has a noticeably calming effect on the digestive system and our general well-being. Researchers have attributed this effect to the quercetin content, a potent anti-inflammatory ability.

Rooibos tea is made by steeping one teaspoon of the herb in a cup of hot water for approximately 3-5 minutes before enjoying its natural sweet taste.

Schisandra Berries (Schisandra chinensis)

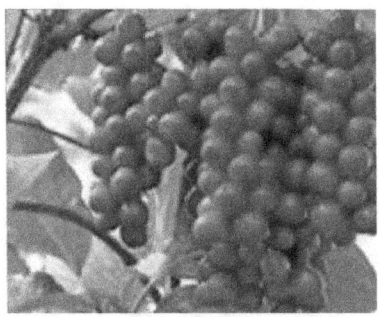

Schisandra (Schisandra chinensis) is an aromatic woody vine and can reach heights of up to 25 feet. Native to China, Schisandra is a member of the Magnoliaceae family. The berries have a sweet, sour, hot, salty and bitter taste and thus are named "Wu Wei Zi" in China which translates to mean, five flavored herb. Since it possesses all five flavors, it is also said to benefit all five of the yin organs: liver, kidneys, heart, lungs and spleen.

This amazing herb holds a top spot in Traditional Chinese Medicine (TCM) due to its superior medicinal benefits which include adaptogenic, antioxidant, anti-fatigue, anti-inflammatory, astringent, cardiotonic, expectorant, immune support, liver protective, mental function and nervine, to name a few.

Organic Schisandra berry powder can be found on-line and mixed in juice, water, smoothie or a tea.

Skullcap (Scutellaria lateriflora)

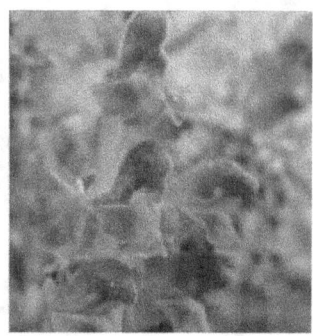

Skullcap, also known as blue skullcap and mad dog skullcap, is a hardy perennial herb of the mint family, Lamiaceae. Although native to North America, it is now widely cultivated in Europe and other areas of the world.

Skullcap is a powerful medicinal herb used in alternative medicine as an anti-inflammatory, antispasmodic, nervine, sedative and strong tonic.

Scientific studies are proving this herb to be a valuable plant in many areas for mental disorders. Skullcap is used in the treatment of a wide range of nervous conditions including epilepsy, insomnia, hysteria, anxiety, delirium tremens, withdrawal from barbiturates and tranquilizers.

A medicinal infusion of the plant is used to promote menstruation, it should not be given to pregnant women since it can induce a miscarriage, and the infusion is also used in the treatment of throat infections. The infusion is given for nervous headaches, neuralgia and in headache arising from incessant coughing, pain, and inducing sleep when necessary, without any unpleasant symptoms following. Skullcap is currently being used as an alternative medicine to treat ADD and a number of nerve disorders.

Skullcap has been used for over two hundred years as a mild relaxant and has long been hailed as an effective therapy for anxiety, nervous tension, and convulsions due to its calming effects on the nervous and musculoskeletal system.

St John's Wort (Hypericum perforatum)

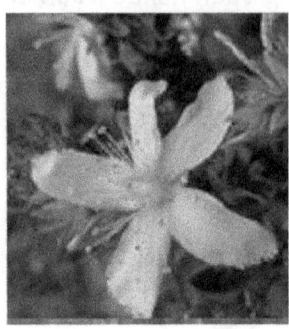

Extracts of St. John's wort exert an antidepressant effect by inhibiting the reuptake of the neurotransmitters including serotonin, norepinephrine and dopamine.

The St. John's wort (Hypericum perforatum) plant has yellow flowers and is considered to be a weed throughout most of the United States. It has been used for medical purposes in other parts of the world for thousands of years.

St. John's wort is very helpful in relieving anxiety as it strengthens and nourishes the nerves.

To make tea, add one to two teaspoons of dried St. John's wort into a cup of boiling water and steep for 10 minutes before using. The recommended dosage of tea is one to two cups daily. Four to six weeks may be necessary in order to notice improvement in symptoms of depression.

Valerian (Valeriana officinalis)

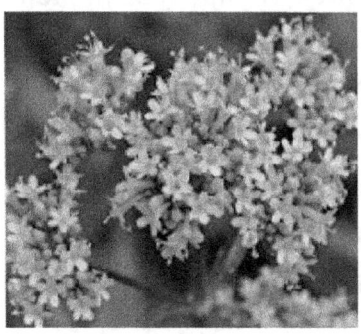

Valerian is a nervine from which medicine is made from its root. Valerian is most commonly used for sleep disorders, especially insomnia, anxiety and nervous restlessness. It is frequently combined with hops, lemon balm, or other herbs that also contain sedative properties. Some people who are trying to withdraw from the use of "sleeping pills" use valerian to help in this respect, allowing them to fall asleep naturally after they have tapered the dose of the sleeping pill.

Although some herbs help reduce anxiety without making you drowsy, while others reduce anxiety and help you sleep, Valerian falls in the latter group. The German government recognizes this fact and has formerly approved this herb as a remedy for sleep disorders, such as insomnia.

Valerian is also used for conditions connected to anxiety and psychological stress including nervous asthma, hysterical states, excitability, and fear of illness (hypochondria), headaches, migraine, and stomach upset. Some people use valerian specifically for depression. It has also been found effective for mild tremors, epilepsy, attention deficit-hyperactivity disorder (ADHD), and chronic fatigue syndrome (CFS).

Valerian is used for muscle and joint pain. Some women use valerian for menstrual cramps and symptoms associated with menopause, including hot flashes and anxiety. Sometimes, valerian is added to bath water as another way to help with restlessness and sleep disorders.

Valerian tea: Boil 1 teaspoon of Valerian powder (or chopped fresh or dried root) in 1 cup of water; let it steep for up to 20 minutes before straining and drinking.

It should be noted that Valerian has a strong odor that some people find offensive and for this reason, in order to obtain the benefits of Valerian, they insist on mixing this herb with lemon balm, mint, chamomile and even honey to make the tea more palatable.

Wormwood (Artemisia absinthium)

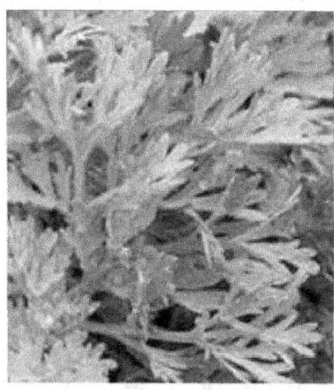

Knowledge of wormwood and its psychoactive properties can be traced back to ancient times. It was the main ingredient of the legendary drink "absinthe" which was invented in 1792 by a French doctor. Intended as medicine, it wound up becoming quite popular as a recreational drink. The effects are said to be narcotic and mildly hallucinogenic.

The plant's scientific name, Artemisia absinthium, stems from its association with the virgin Greek goddess Artemis, who held it and other species of Artemisia sacred.

Wormwood is an easy perennial to grow, requiring little to no maintenance. I've kept a Wormwood garden for years in my backyard, as the plant will survive winter after winter, growing back even more vigorously and aromatic the next year.

All parts of the plant above the ground are psychoactive and contain the main alkaloid known as thujone, as well as the bitter material known as absinthum; wormwood essential oil is very rich in thujone. Because of the presence of thujone, an extremely potent psychoactive substance, absinthe liquor is much stronger than other types of liquors, therefore producing very different effects. There are frequent reports that while on absinthe; one experiences a profound sense of euphoria, aphrodisiac sensations, hallucinations and a feeling of floating.

Dried wormwood herbage can be smoked alone or as part of a smoking blend. It is also used as incense, generally in smudge bundles. Fresh or dried wormwood herbage can also be added to boiling water and allowed to steep for five minutes. One gram of dried leaves in a cup of hot water corresponds to a single medicinal dose.

Due to the tea's bitter taste which is mostly unavoidable, try adding peppermint leaves or anise to reduce the bitterness taste.

To make "absinthe", soak 40 grams (1 ½ oz.) of wormwood for a couple of weeks in ½ jar of liquor. After this time, strain the plant material and discard. The drink is now ready to enjoy. It is advisable to take one small glass at first and wait for the effects prior to taking more.

Closing Remarks

Stress is at the root of many health conditions. When the body is stressed, our capacity to adapt is greatly reduced, which can have detrimental effects on the immune and nervous system. Optimizing adrenal gland function is essential in combating stress.

The calming herbs discussed in this book can be found in a supplement form. However, it is to your advantage to consume these herbs, in a tea. Many of these herbs are hardy and can be grown in your garden or in a pot on your balcony or deck, such as lemon balm, lavender etc.

Among traditional medicine, adaptogenic herbs are used worldwide for stress relief and revitalization of health, including Ayurveda, Traditional Chinese Medicine as well as in Africa, South America and Europe. Conventional or allopathic medicine in North America focuses primarily on the treatment of specific illnesses rather than preventative care and maintenance of overall health. This has proved to be very costly and ineffective.

About the Author

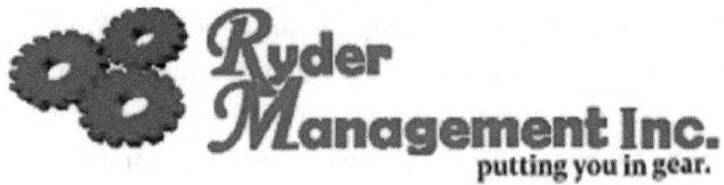

Located in London, Canada, Ryder Management Inc is a publisher whose primary focus is on natural healing remedies.

Rydermgt acts as an umbrella organization for a number of independent authors with common and like goals of helping others achieve optimal health naturally.

If you enjoyed this book, please tell others; otherwise please tell us!

Other Kindle books written by Ryder Management Inc

Please see other Kindle books written by Ryder Management Inc authors at our author page on amazon.com by clicking or copying the following link:

http://www.amazon.com/Ryder-Management-Inc./e/B00ICGMCRS

Ryder Management Inc also has a website at rydermanagement.ca

Our email address is info@rydermanagement.ca

References and Sources

Truly Organic Foods: http://www.trulyorganicfoods.com/

Mountain Rose Herbs: www.mountainroseherbs.com

US Plant Database:
http://plants.usda.gov/core/profile?symbol=VEHA2

Judy's Organic Herbs "Herbs with Spirit": www.earthmedicine.ca